Vegan Quotes

NOTEBOOK

ISBN 978-1-365-28331-4

"Don't wait for a better world. Start now to create a world of harmony and peace. It is up to you, and it always has been. You may even find the solution at the end of your fork."

SHARON GANNON

4

"A man can live and be healthy without killing animals for food; therefore, if he eats meat, he participates in taking animal life merely for the sake of his appetite. And to act so is immoral."

LEO TOLSTOY

"One farmer says to me, 'You cannot live on vegetable food solely, for it furnishes nothing to make the bones with;' and so he religiously devotes a part of his day to supplying himself with the raw material of bones; walking all the while he talks behind his oxen, which, with vegetable-made bones, jerk him and his lumbering plow along in spite of every obstacle."

HENRY DAVID THOREAU

"Refrain at all times from such foods as cannot
be procured without violence and oppression."
THOMAS TRYON

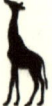

"Some people think the plant-based, whole-foods diet is
extreme. Half a million people a year will have their chests
opened up and a vein taken from their leg and sewn onto their
coronary artery. Some people would call that extreme."
DR. CALDWELL ESSELSTYN

"My refusing to eat meat occasioned inconveniency,
and I have been frequently chided for my singularity.
But my light repast allows for greater progress, for
greater clearness of head and quicker comprehension."
BENJAMIN FRANKLIN

"After all the information I gathered about the mistreatment of animals, I couldn't continue to eat meat. The more I was aware of, the harder and harder it was to do."
LIAM HEMSWORTH

"I believe I am not interested to know whether vivisection produces results that are profitable to the human race or doesn't. To know that the results are profitable to the race would not remove my hostility to it. The pains which it inflicts upon unconsenting animals is the basis of my enmity towards it, and it is to me sufficient justification of the enmity without looking further."

MARK TWAIN

"The human body has no more need for cows' milk than
it does for dogs' milk, horses' milk, or giraffes' milk."
MICHAEL KLAPER

"Perhaps in the back of our minds we already understand, without all the science I've discussed, that something terribly wrong is happening. Our sustenance now comes from misery. We know that if someone offers to show us a film on how our meat is produced, it will be a horror film. We perhaps know more than we care to admit, keeping it down in the dark places of our memory—disavowed. When we eat factory-farmed meat we live, literally, on tortured flesh. Increasingly, that tortured flesh is becoming our own."

JONATHAN SAFRAN

"We all love animals. Why do we
call some 'pets' and others 'dinner'?"
K.D. LANG

"Whenever people say 'We mustn't be sentimental'
you can take it they are about to do something
cruel. And if they add 'We must be realistic' they
mean they are going to make money out of it."
BRIGID BROPHY

"We consume the carcasses of creatures of like
appetites, passions and organs with our own, and fill the
slaughterhouses daily with screams of pain and fear."
ROBERT LOUIS STEVENSON

"I made the choice to be vegan because I will not eat (or wear, or use) anything that could have an emotional response to its death or captivity. I can well imagine what that must feel like for our non-human friends—the fear, the terror, the pain— and I will not cause such suffering to a fellow living being."

RAI AREN

"Luckily we know that you can get your protein source from many different ways, you can get it through vegetables if you are a vegetarian. I have seen many body builders that are vegetarian and they get strong and healthy."
ARNOLD SCHWARZENEGGER

"Being vegan is easy. Are there social pressures that encourage you to continue to eat, wear, and use animal products? Of course there are. But in a patriarchal, racist, homophobic, and ableist society, there are social pressures to participate and engage in sexism, racism, homophobia, and ableism. At some point, you have to decide who you are and what matters morally to you. And once you decide that you regard victimizing vulnerable nonhumans is not morally acceptable, it is easy to go and stay vegan."

GARY L. FRANCIONE

"Thou should eat to live; not live to eat."
SOCRATES

"Veganism is not about giving anything up or losing anything; it is about gaining the peace within yourself that comes from embracing nonviolence and refusing to participate in the exploitation of the vulnerable."

GARY L. FRANCIONE

"If you don't like seeing pictures of violence
towards animals being posted, you need to
help stop the violence, not the pictures."
JOHNNY DEPP

"Elsewhere the paper notes that vegetarians and vegans (including athletes) 'meet and exceed requirements' for protein. And, to render the whole we-should-worry-about-getting-enough-protein-and-therefore-eat-meat idea even more useless, other data suggests that excess animal protein intake is linked with osteoporosis, kidney disease, calcium stones in the urinary tract, and some cancers. Despite some persistent confusion, it is clear that vegetarians and vegans tend to have more optimal protein consumption than omnivores."

JONATHAN SAFRAN

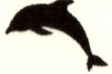

"How can people spend this Christmas season talking
of 'peace on earth' and 'love' and then sit down to
devour someone who never knew love or peace?"
JUDY STEPHENS SNOOK

"The sixteen hundred dairies in California's Central Valley alone produce more waste than a city of twenty-one million people—that's more than the populations of London, New York, and Chicago combined."
GENE BAUR

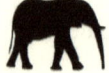

"Suffering is suffering. It is always ugly. It is always unwelcome. It always needs to be stopped. There are no exceptions. A person with the capacity but not the inclination to cease suffering is morally incomplete."
MIRKO BAGARIC

"Love animals: God has given them the rudiments of thought and joy untroubled. Do not trouble their joy, don't harass them, don't deprive them of their happiness, don't work against God's intent. Man, do not pride yourself on superiority to animals; they are without sin, and you, with your greatness, defile the earth by your appearance on it, and leave the traces of your foulness after you—alas, it is true of almost every one of us!"

FYODOR DOSTOYEVSKI

"A hundred and fifty years ago, they would have thought you were absurd if you advocated for the end of slavery. A hundred years ago, they would have laughed at you for suggesting that women should have the right to vote. Fifty years ago, they would object to the idea of African Americans receiving equal rights under the law. Twenty-five years ago they would have called you a pervert if you advocated for gay rights. They laugh at us now for suggesting that animal slavery be ended. Some day they won't be laughing."

GARY SMITH

"Do you know why most survivors of the
Holocaust are vegan? It's because they know
what it's like to be treated like an animal."
CHUCK PALAHNIUK

"We have enslaved the rest of animal creation and have treated our distant cousins in fur and feathers so badly that beyond doubt, if they were to formulate a religion, they would depict the Devil in human form."
WILLIAM RALPH INGE

"I choose not to make a graveyard of my body
for the rotting corpses of dead animals."
GEORGE BERNARD SHAW

"People often say that humans have always eaten animals, as if this is a justification for continuing to the practice. According to this logic, we should not try to prevent people from murdering other people, since this has also been done since the earliest of times."

ISAAC BASHEVIS SINGER

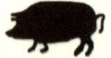

"It was all so very businesslike that one watched it fascinated. It was pork-making by machinery, pork-making by applied mathematics. And yet somehow the most matter-of-fact person could not help thinking of the hogs; they were so innocent, they came so very trustingly; and they were so very human in their protests—and so perfectly within their rights! They had done nothing to deserve it; and it was adding insult to injury, as the thing was done here, swinging them up in this cold-blooded, impersonal way, without pretence at apology, without the homage of a tear."

UPTON SINCLAIR

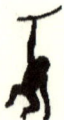

"My perspective of veganism was most affected by
learning that the veal calf is a by-product of dairying, and
that in essence there is a slice of veal in every glass of what
I had thought was an innocuous white liquid—milk."

RYNN BERRY

"Violence begins with the fork."
MOHANDAS GANDHI

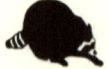

"As long as people will shed the blood of innocent creatures there can be no peace, no liberty, no harmony between people. Slaughter and justice cannot dwell together."
ISAAC BASHEVIS SINGER

"The path of the norm is the path of least resistance; it is the route we take when we're on auto-pilot and don't even realize we're following a course of action that we haven't consciously chosen. Most people who eat meat have no idea that they're behaving in accordance with the tenets of a system that has defined many of their values, preferences, and behaviors. What they call 'free choice' is, in fact, the result of a narrowly obstructed set of options that have been chosen for them. They don't realize, for instance, that they have been taught to value human life so far above certain forms of nonhuman life that it seems appropriate for their taste preferences to supersede other species' preference for survival."

MELANIE JOY

"We patronize them for their incompleteness, for their tragic fate for having taken form so far below ourselves. And therein do we err. For the animal shall not be measured by man. In a world older and more complete than ours, they move finished and complete, gifted with the extension of the senses we have lost or never attained, living by voices we shall never hear. They are not brethren, they are not underlings: they are other nations, caught with ourselves in the net of life and time, fellow prisoners of the splendour and travail of the earth."

HENRY BESTON

"Being vegetarian here also means that we do not consume dairy
and egg products, because they are products of the meat industry.
If we stop consuming, they will stop producing. Only collective
awakening can create enough determination for action."

THÍCH NHAT HANH

"The worst sin toward our fellow creatures is not to hate them,
but to be indifferent to them: that's the essence of inhumanity."
GEORGE BERNARD SHAW

"Poor animals, how jealously they guard their bodies, for to us is merely an evening's meal, but to them is life itself."
T. CASEY BRENNAN

"Take away Love and our earth is a tomb."
ROBERT BROWNING

"There is something about veganism that is not easy, but the difficulty is not inherent in veganism, but in our culture."
WILL TUTTLE

"A man is ethical only when life, as such, is sacred to him, that of plants and animals as that of his fellow men, and when he devotes himself helpfully to all life that is in need of help."
ALBERT SCHWEITZER

"Our economic order is tightly woven around the exploitation of animals, and while it may seem easy to dismiss concern about animals as the soft-headed mental masturbation of people who really don't understand oppression and the depths of actual human misery, I hope to get you to think differently about suffering and pain, to convince you that animals matter, and to argue that anyone serious about ending domination and hierarchy needs to think critically about bringing animals into consideration."

BOB TORRES

"An animal's eyes have the power to speak a great language."
MARTIN BUBER

"If you don't take care of this the most magnificent machine
that you will ever be given ... where are you going to live?"
KARYN CALABRESE

"The human spirit is not dead. It lives on in secret. ... It has come to believe that compassion, in which all ethics must take root, can only attain its full breadth and depth if it embraces all living creatures and does not limit itself to mankind."
ALBERT SCHWEITZER

"Personal purity isn't really the issue. Not supporting animal abuse—and persuading others not to support it—is."
PETER SINGER

"One should not kill a living being, nor cause it to be killed, nor should one incite another to kill. Do not injure any being, either strong or weak, in the world."

BUDDHA

"Go to the meat market of a Saturday night and see the crowds of live bipeds staring up at the long rows of dead quadrupeds. Does not that sight take a tooth out of the cannibal's jaw? Cannibals? Who is not a cannibal? I tell you it will be more tolerable for the Fejee that salted down a lean missionary in his cellar against a coming famine; it will be more tolerable for that provident Fejee, I say, in the day of judgement, than for thee, civilized and enlightened gourmand, who nailest geese to the ground and feasteth on their bloated livers in thy paté-de-foie-gras."

HERMAN MELVILLE

"The thinking man must oppose all cruel customs no matter how deeply rooted in tradition and surrounded by a halo. When we have a choice, we must avoid bringing torment and injury into the life of another, even the lowliest creature; to do so is to renounce our manhood and shoulder a guilt which nothing justifies."

ALBERT SCHWEITZER

"Human beings have capitalized on the silence of animals,
just as certain human beings have historically imposed
silence on certain other human beings by denying slaves
the right to literacy, denying women the right to own
property, and denying both the right to vote."
GARY STEINER

"It is more important to prevent animal suffering,
rather than sit to contemplate the evils of the
universe praying in the company of priests."
BUDDHA

"Nobody can possibly be so hungry that they need to
take a life in order to feel satisfied—they don't after all,
take a human life, so why take the life of an animal?
Both are conscious beings with the same determination
to survive. It is habit, and laziness and nothing else."
MORRISSEY

"I will not kill or hurt any living creature
needlessly, nor destroy any beautiful thing, but will
strive to save and comfort all gentle life, and guard
and perfect all natural beauty upon the earth."
JOHN RUSKIN

"This for many people is what is most offensive about hunting—to some, disgusting: that it encourages, or allows, us not only to kill but to take a certain pleasure in killing. It's not as though the rest of us don't countenance the killing of tens of millions of animals every year. Yet for some reason we feel more comfortable with the mechanical killing practiced, out of view and without emotion, by industrial agriculture."

MICHAEL POLLAN

"We cannot have peace among men whose hearts
find delight in killing any living creature."
RACHEL CARSON

"If your meals consistently revolve around corpse multiple
times daily, you might become one sooner than you planned."
KRIS CARR

"For as long as men massacre animals, they will kill each other. Indeed, he who sows the seed of murder and pain cannot reap joy and love."
PYTHAGORAS

"I am not well-versed in theory, but in my view, the cow deserves her life. As does the ram. As does the ladybug. As does the elephant. As do the fish, and the dog and the bee; as do other sentient beings. I will always be in favor of veganism as a minimum because I believe that sentient beings have a right not to be used as someone else's property. They ask us to be brave for them, to be clear for them, and I see no other acceptable choice but to advocate veganism. If these statements make me a fundamentalist, then I will sew a scarlet F on my jacket so that all may know I'm fundamentally in favor of nonviolence; may they bury me in it so that all will know where I stood."

VINCENT J. GUIHAN

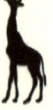

"Isn't man an amazing animal? He kills wildlife—birds, kangaroos, deer, all kinds
of cats, coyotes, beavers, groundhogs, mice, foxes and dingoes—by the million
in order to protect his domestic animals and their feed. Then he kills domestic
animals by the billion and eats them. This in turn kills man by the million, because
eating all those animals leads to degenerative—and fatal—health conditions like
heart disease, kidney disease, and cancer. So then man tortures and kills millions
more animals to look for cures for these diseases. Elsewhere, millions of other
human beings are being killed by hunger and malnutrition because food they
could eat is being used to fatten domestic animals. Meanwhile, some people are
dying of sad laughter at the absurdity of man, who kills so easily and so violently,
and once a year, sends out cards praying for Peace on Earth."

C. DAVID COATS

"Cruelty to animals is an enormous injustice; so is expecting those on the lowest rung of the economic ladder to do the dangerous, soul-numbing work of slaughtering sentient beings on our behalf."
VICTORIA MORAN

"But for the sake of some little mouthful of flesh we deprive a soul of the sun and light, and of that proportion of life and time it had been born into the world to enjoy."

PLUTARCH

"I have no doubt that it is a part of the destiny of the human race, in its gradual improvement, to leave off eating animals, as surely as the savage tribes have left off eating each other."
HENRY DAVID THOREAU

"The time will come when men such as I will look upon the
murder of animals as they now look upon the murder of men."
LEONARDO DA VINCI

"I don't believe vegans (or vegetarians) who still get their (packaged, preservative/ chemical-ridden) food from industrial food systems have any righteous ground to stand on, nor do I think a deep look at the sentient life of plants or the true environmental impact of agriculture permits them any comfortable distance from cruelty. Everything in this world eats something else to survive, and that something else, whether running on blood or chlorophyll, would always rather continue to live rather than become sustenance for another. No animal wants to be penned up and milked, or caged and harvested, and you've never seen plants growing in regimented lines of their own accord."
BRIAN AWEHALI

"Recognize meat for what it really is: the antibiotic-
and pesticide-laden corpse of a tortured animal."
INGRID NEWKIRK

"The vegan lifestyle is a compassionate way
to live that supports life, supports fairness
and equality, and promotes freedom."
ROBERT CHEEKE

"Non-violence leads to the highest ethics, which
is the goal of all evolution. Until we stop harming
all other living beings, we are still savages."
THOMAS EDISON

"Becoming vegan is the most important and direct change we
can immediately make to save the planet and its species."
CHRIS HEDGES

"Could you look an animal in the eyes and say to it, 'My
appetite is more important than your suffering'?"
MOBY

"Without pushing an agenda (okay, maybe I've pushed a bit), I've spread a little veganism wherever I've gone. I've become friends with chefs at the meatiest restaurants you can imagine, and shown them a few things that opened their minds (and their menus) to vegan options. It's easy to be convincing when the food is delicious. It doesn't feel like a sacrifice—it feels like a step up."

TAL RONNEN

"Until one has loved an animal, a part
of one's soul remains unawakened."
ANATOLE FRANCE

"In California, the state's huge dairy herd produces twenty-seven million tons of manure a year, the particulates and vapors from which have helped to make air quality in the agriculturally intensive San Joaquin Valley worse than it is Los Angeles."
PAUL ROBERTS

"If you don't want to be beaten, imprisoned, mutilated, killed or tortured then you shouldn't condone such behaviour towards anyone, be they human or not."
MOBY

"I remember looking at the fear in her eyes. How could someone be so cruel? I thought as the hens cried. When will people realize that other animals have just as much the right as we do."
ZOE ROSENBERG

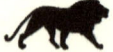

"We do not need to eat animals, wear animals, or use
animals for entertainment purposes, and our only defence
of these uses is our pleasure, amusement, and convenience."
GARY L. FRANCIONE

"We know we cannot be kind to animals until we stop exploiting them — exploiting animals in the name of science, exploiting animals in the name of sport, exploiting animals in the name of fashion, and yes, exploiting animals in the name of food."
CÉSAR CHÁVEZ

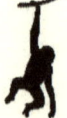

"Intellectually, human beings and animals may be different,
but it's pretty obvious that animals have a rich emotional
life and that they feel joy and pain. It's easy to forget the
connection between a hamburger and the cow it came from.
But I forced myself to acknowledge the fact that every time I
ate a hamburger, a cow had ceased to breathe."

MOBY

"I am very proud of the fact that twenty years on people tell me they became a vegetarian as a result of 'Meat Is Murder.' I think that is quite literally rock music changing someone's life—it's certainly changing the life of animals. It is one of the things I am most proud of."
JOHNNY MARR

"I hold that the more helpless a creature, the more entitled
it is to protection by man from the cruelty of man."
MOHANDAS GANDHI

"I do not see any reason why animals should be slaughtered to serve as human diet when there are so many substitutes. After all, man can live without meat. It is only some carnivorous animals that have to subsist on flesh. Killing animals for sport, for pleasure, for adventures, and for hides and furs is a phenomenon which is at once disgusting and distressing. There is no justification in indulging in such acts of brutality. ... Life is as dear to a mute creature as it is to a man. Just as one wants happiness and fears pain, just as one wants to live and not to die, so do other creatures."

THE DALAI LAMA

"I became a vegan the day I watched a video of a calf being born on a factory farm. The baby was dragged away from his mother before he hit the ground. The helpless calf strained its head backwards to find his mother. The mother bolted after her son and exploded into a rage when the rancher slammed the gate on her. She wailed the saddest noise I'd ever heard an animal make, and then thrashed and ... dug into the ground, burying her face in the muddy placenta. I had no idea what was happening respecting brain chemistry, animal instinct, or whatever. I just knew that this was deeply wrong. I just knew that such suffering could never be worth the taste of milk and veal. I empathized with the cow and the calf and, in so doing, my life changed."

JAMES MCWILLIAMS

"Humans—who enslave, castrate, experiment on, and fillet other animals—have had an understandable penchant for pretending animals do not feel pain. A sharp distinction between humans and 'animals' is essential if we are to bend them to our will, make them work for us, wear them, eat them–without any disquieting tinges of guilt or regret. It is unseemly of us, who often behave so unfeelingly toward other animals, to contend that only humans can suffer. The behavior of other animals renders such pretensions specious. They are just too much like us."

CARL SAGAN

"In fact, if one person is unkind to an animal it is considered to be cruelty, but where a lot of people are unkind to animals, especially in the name of commerce, the cruelty is condoned and, once large sums of money are at stake, will be defended to the last by otherwise intelligent people."

RUTH HARRISON

www.ingramcontent.com/pod-product-compliance
Lightning Source LLC
Chambersburg PA
CBHW020431290526
45785CB00002B/791